Permanently Beat Bacterial Vaginosis

Proven 3 Day Cure for Bacterial Vaginosis Freedom, Natural Treatment That Will Prevent Recurring Infection and Vaginal Odor

Caroline D. Greene

Published by Women's Republic

Atlanta, Georgia USA

WOMEN'S
Republic

ISBN 978-1-4839-0316-3

What Our Readers Are Saying

Words from the Author

Just saying the name of this disease out loud can make one feel uncomfortable and maybe a little bit scared. However, it's not as dangerous as it sounds and it's quite treatable. But to get the correct treatment you first have to be diagnosed and when it comes to this particular condition, that can often be the tricky part.

I wrote this book to help women identify the symptoms of this illness by themselves and so enable them to seek help as soon as they begin to suspect they may have BV. I've been researching women health topics for years, during which time I came to realize that one of the most important problems in dealing with these issues is that a lot of them are never openly discussed. Not talking about them doesn't help anyone; not the sick person and not the healthy ones who are unknowingly at risk. People need to know, and my personal mission is to bring these issues to the forefront.

Bacterial Vaginosis is a surprisingly common illness, and in the pages of this book I explain in detail all the whats and the whys, and how it can affect your life if left untreated. Looks a lot of time can deceive, and so can symptoms. By reading this guide you'll be arm yourself with the facts, and should you find yourself faced with BV, beat the disease and get back to living a normal, healthy life.

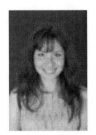

Caroline D. Greene

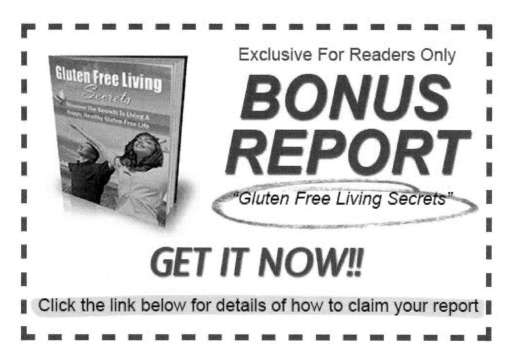

Exclusive Bonus Download: Gluten Free Living Secrets

Are you sick and tired of trying every weight loss program out there and failing to see results? Or are you frustrated with not feeling as energetic as you used to despite what you eat? Perhaps you always seem to have a bit of a "dodgy stomach" and indigestion seems to be a regular part of your life?

There's nothing worse than sitting down to a nice big plate of pasta and enjoying your meal only to be met with a growling stomach and the inevitable rush to the toilet.

It's that bloated feeling you get after eating a piece of bread that just "doesn't seem right" . Almost as if you've eaten something poisonous.

Gluten Free Living Secrets is a complete resource that will tell you everything you need to know about the dangers of eating gluten and how to go about transitioning yourself and your family to a life free of this dangerous substance.

Here's just a taste of what you will discover inside Gluten Free Living Secrets:

- What foods you should focus on when first switching to a gluten-free diet

- The 9 grains that are safe and gluten-free

- The truth about whether you can eat pasta on a gluten-free diet

- What you should know to determine if you have Celiac Disease

- and that's not all...

- Why you may want to consider eliminating gluten from your child's diet

- The top 10 reasons to go gluten-free

- How to transform your pantry to be gluten-free

- A list of essential gluten-free shopping tips

- How to keep your kids happy around their gluten-eating friends

- Tips on staying gluten-free when eating out

Go to the end of this book for the download link for this Bonus

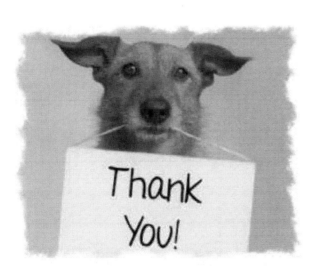

Thank you for downloading my book. Please REVIEW this book on Amazon. I need your feedback to make the next version better. Thank you so much!

Books by This Author

<u>Permanently Beat Bacterial Vaginosis</u>

<u>Permanently Beat Yeast Infection & Candida</u>

<u>Permanently Beat Urinary Tract Infections</u>

<u>Permanently Beat Hypothyroidism Naturally</u>

<u>Permanently Beat PCOS</u>

<u>The Permanently Beat PCOS Diet & Exercise Shortcuts</u>

<u>The Permanently Beat Hypothyroidism Diet & Exercise Shortcuts</u>

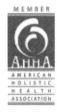

Table of Content

Disclaimer

While all attempts have been made to provide effective, verifiable information in this Book, neither the Author nor Publisher assumes any responsibility for errors, inaccuracies, or omissions. Any slights of people or organizations are unintentional.

This Book is not a source of medical information, and it should not be regarded as such. This publication is designed to provide accurate and authoritative information in regard to the subject matter covered. It is sold with the understanding that the publisher is not engaged in rendering a medical service. As with any medical advice, the reader is strongly encouraged to seek professional medical advice before taking action.

Chapter 1: Understanding Bacterial Vaginosis

If you have come to this book then you are probably suffering from chronic bacterial vaginosis .But do you really understand what it is? You may recognize it when you are feeling itchy, unclean and even smelly but you may not know much more than that about it. Bacterial vaginosis is an infection in your vagina that leaves you not only in discomfort but also in embarrassment. It can keep you from doing the things you enjoy and can be particularly difficult to shake it off.

A doctor will most likely prescribe you antibiotics to treat the infection but it will only give you relief for a short time (not to mention, you will then have to deal with the potential side effects from the antibiotics, too.) Before you know it, bacterial vaginosis is back and wreaking havoc on your body and life. Whenever a medical condition has "osis" at the end of it, it indicates that the condition is chronic and persistent; i.e. it will keep coming back.

If you don't know what you are doing, you can battle bacterial vaginosis for many, many years. This is a very difficult infection to get rid of permanently. Often, just when you think it has finally cleared up, its nasty symptoms start to appear again. So what do you do? Give up and accept it as fate? It is an upsetting situation, but you have come this far and can't give up now! The good news is that there is a way to get rid of bacterial vaginosis once and for all - and it does NOT include antibiotics or any other prescribed medicine. But before you can get rid of it for good, you have to understand what it really is.

How Do You Get It?

There is a reason for every illness and every infection that your body can become inflicted with. Unfortunately, sometimes the specifics aren't yet completely understood. When it comes to developing a bacterial vaginosis infection, scientists are not entirely sure why or how it happens but they do know this: Bacterial vaginosis occurs when there is an imbalance of the bacteria that normally lives in the vagina. Not all bacteria are bad; in fact, our bodies need certain levels of it in order to stay healthy. When our normal levels of healthy bacteria decrease, it makes are bodies susceptible to "bad" bacteria moving in, and overcoming the good. When this happens, we end up with a bacterial infection.

Although bacterial vaginosis is often developed after having sex with a new man, it is technically not considered a sexually transmitted infection; because it doesn't only develop after sex. In fact, many women are too embarrassed to tell their doctor about their symptoms because they mistakenly think it can only be from sexual intercourse. Worried their doctors will judge them for being promiscuous, they say nothing and the infection rages unchecked. The truth is, even if you have never had sex before, you can still end up with bacterial vaginosis.

Bacterial vaginosis is actually the most common culprit behind vaginal infection. It is important to distinguish the difference between bacterial vaginosis, yeast infection and trichomoniasis. Though they may share similar symptoms; bacterial vaginosis is caused by bacteria, while yeast infections and trichomoiasis are not. Because it is bacterially based, bacterial vaginosis can come and go on a chronic basis.

What Are the Symptoms?

Though there are very typical symptoms of bacterial vaginosis; some women who are tested positive to have it, never have any symptoms at all. In fact as much as half, half of the women who have it don't even realize they have it. If you have no symptoms, then there is no reason to treat it, though you may want to adjust your lifestyle to keep it from coming back, because next time it could present symptoms. And believe me, you do not want to have to deal with these awful symptoms.

The most common symptoms of bacterial vaginosis are:

Vaginal discharge that is watery or thin; grey or white; or has a strong, fishy smell

Vaginal discharge is by the by far the most common symptom of bacterial vaginosis. Many women describe the discharge as leaving them with a slimy feeling and that they never can feel clean, no matter how much they clean their vaginal area. Even worse, the fishy smell is so strong that they feel embarrassed and then avoid having sex with their partner in fear that he will smell it too, and be grossed out. In fact, if you do have sex while you have this infection, the fishy smell can intensify both during and after sex.

Burning feeling while urinating

As soon as you begin to urinate, you feel a burning pain inside your vagina that is enough to make you want to stop.

Itchiness around the outside of your vagina

You almost constantly feel the urge to scratch the outside area of your vagina. Especially if you are wearing underwear or pants that are tight against you. The urge to itch is so strong that it is almost impossible to resist.

Pain during sex

Upon penetration during sex, you will feel abnormal vaginal pain. The pain will be alleviated upon withdrawal.

NOTE: *It is important to realize that these symptoms are not only true of bacterial vaginosis but also of other vaginal infections including many sexually transmitted diseases and vaginally transmitted infections.* Because of this, if you suspect you have a bacterial vaginosis infection, particularly if it is the first time for you, you *should visit your doctor to confirm the diagnosis.* Your doctor can test you for other STDs and infections to rule them out. If it is something else, you may require different treatment or else the disease or infection can spread and cause a lot of damage including infertility.

What Increases My Risk of Getting it?

Your chance of developing it is greatly increased if you have multiple sex partners. Also, smoking can increase your risk of developing it. Some hygiene products such as douches have been linked to an increased risk of bacterial vaginosis.

With that being said, there is a good chance that you could develop bacterial vaginosis at some point in your life. In fact, the CDC (Centre for Disease Control) estimates that roughly 16% of American women suffer from bacterial vaginosis. While that percentage may not seem that high, realize that this statistic translates to roughly 25 million women,in the US alone.

While virtually any woman can get bacterial vaginosis, there are certain things that increase your chances:

Using douches

Douches were once acceptable methods of cleaning your vagina but over the years they have become almost taboo. Vaginal tissue is very sensitive; any forced water or solution can cause an infection.

Bathing with scented, perfumed or antiseptic liquids, bubble baths or soaps.

If you have ever put regular soap near your vaginal opening before, you probably noticed the burning sensation it caused. Again, vaginal tissue is sensitive. Using anything that is scented or has some sort of chemical (even if the label says it is for sensitive areas) can cause infection. Stick to non-scented soaps and skip soaking in anything other than pure water.

Having a new sex partner

Having sex with someone new can leave you with an infection because any infection that they may have will be passed to you. This is why it is especially important to pay attention to any symptoms that may arise shortly after you begin a new sexual relationship.

Having multiple sex partners

Having sex with multiple people increases your chances of catching many infections and diseases, including bacterial vaginosis. You are introducing your body, particularly your vagina, to many different varieties of bacteria. It is easy for your natural bacteria to be overcome by all these new bacteria.

Smoking

Smoking increases your risks of developing many diseases and infections and bacterial vaginosis is no different. When you smoke a cigarette, you are inhaling all manner of carcinogens and other unhealthy chemicals. These cannot only lower your overall immunity but can also kill healthy bacteria that fight the bad bacteria.

Using an IUD

It's only common sense that having a foreign object in your body can cause some internal problems. One of these problems is infection. If you recently had an IUD inserted and you are suddenly having fishy discharge or itching, you may be better off having it removed; instead of dealing with bacterial vaginosis over and over again.

Using Vaginal Cleaners

Similar to the above points about scented soaps, when you use anything other than plain water to clean or deodorize your vagina, you are leaving yourself open to infection.

Using strong detergent for your underwear

Not only can strong detergent lingering on your underwear irritate the outside of your vagina, but it can also irritate you inside of your vagina. This can certainly imbalance your bacterial level and leave you with an infection.

Birth Control

Whether it's the pill, patch or shot, anything that increases your estrogen levels can leave you with a vaginal infection. While birth control should not entirely be avoided, but you should treat it as any other medicine and make sure that you are taking the proper precautions. (This will be discussed in detail in a later in the book)

Pregnancy

Pregnancy changes a lot of things in your body. The combination of the increased hormones and the other changes your body goes through can greatly affect your bacterial level leaving you extra susceptible to vaginal infection.

Diabetes

It may sound strange, but if you have diabetes, you are at an increased risk of developing bacterial vaginosis. This is most likely due to the medications that you must take in order to control your diabetes and your insulin/blood sugar levels. While you can't get rid of your diabetes, you can take the proper precautions to keep yourself from getting bacterial vaginosis.

While you can get bacterial vaginosis from having sex, you cannot get it from using the same toilet, bedding or swimming pools that someone with bacterial vaginosis has used. You cannot catch the infection from someone else who has it except through sexual intercourse. However, you can develop it on your own without having any contact with the infection at all.

Could it Be Toxins?

Our bodies are intricate machines. They are developed to do everything possible to keep us alive. We are equipped to fight off infection with our own healthy bacteria and white blood cells. We get fevers to fight off infections, and use bowel movements, urination and sweat to rid our bodies of many toxins. After all, this is what it is designed to do.

But what happens if our bodies are on toxin intake overload? These days the human body is subject to many more toxins than it has ever been before in previous years. A prime example of this is the increase of cancer and the development of new types of infections seemingly every day. Everywhere we turn, there are toxins. We may not be able to see them and they may be hiding in places we wouldn't expect, but they are there.

Environmental Toxins

The air we breathe isn't the same as it used to be. Within the air these days are dozens of other components and chemicals. These chemicals are pumped out of factories, vehicles and many more places. You have heard what they are doing to the ozone layer - do you ever wonder if they are doing the same to our bodies?

Well, the fact is that they are! We may not have much control of the environment around us, but we do have control over what products we use ourselves. Pick natural products when you can and live the healthiest lifestyle possible.

Toxins in Our Food

We used to have simple foods made of pure ingredients. Nowadays, even the simplest food is packed with several ingredients - some of which you can't even pronounce. And if you don't make a habit of checking the ingredient list, you probably wouldn't even know that they were in there in the first place. Among the worst toxins that we consume on a regular basis are preservatives. These are the compounds used to make food last on the shelf without going bad.

Have you ever heard that a Twinkie never goes bad? Well, that is probably an exaggeration, but it is based on a fact. The amount of preservatives used in a Twinkie makes it keep its consistency and quality for at least a few years. So basically if you buy a Twinkie today and keep it in its original packaging, you may be able to eat it two years from now. What do you think would happen if you ate that Twinkie? Would any part of it remain in you two years from now? Common sense tells you that there is something wrong with putting this type of thing in your body.

If we are consuming more toxins than our bodies can fight, our bacteria levels will become imbalanced. The bad bacteria will overcome the good and infection will run rampant. Even worse, restoring your body's natural, good bacteria level will be difficult if you continue consuming toxins.

How do we avoid consuming all these extra toxins? By taking it back to basics. Eating fresh food is the best way to avoid many of these toxins and help maintain a natural bacterial balance. This may not completely eliminate or keep you free from bacterial vaginosis on its own but it will certainly make an impact.

Chapter Wrap-Up

At this point, you should have a general understanding of bacterial vaginosis. You know what exactly it is; the many factors that can increase your chances of developing it; the most common symptoms; and even have an insight into why there is such an increase of infection these days.

If after reading this chapter, you realize that you, too, like millions of other women suffer from bacterial vaginosis, then you know that it is not something that you should have to live with. If you want the intense itching, and the uncomfortable and embarrassing discharge gone then you have to be proactive about it. If you do nothing, hoping it will go away; it will continue to linger. On the other hand, you cannot simply rely on your doctor to prescribe you medicine to get rid of it without addressing the underlying cause, because it will invariably come back again and again.

Don't worry - though it may seem like it, the situation is not hopeless. You can live a life free of the restraints that bacterial vaginosis can have over you. Reading this book is the first step towards getting rid of bacterial vaginosis and keeping it away for good.

The following chapters will guide you through every aspect of properly eradicating bacterial vaginosis without having to rely on prescription drugs. So if you are ready to kick those symptoms to the curb once and for all; and take a fresh step into your new life, free of the embarrassment and discomfort that bacterial vaginosis has subjected you to; then let's get right into the next chapter.

Chapter 2: The Negative Impact It Has On Your Life

There's no denying it: bacterial vaginosis can ruin every aspect of your life. If you have spent just one day with this infection, then you know how it can become a real thorn in your side. Besides that irritation, discomfort and embarrassment, do you know what else bacterial vaginosis can do to your life?

Many people underestimate the power that a seemingly "simple" infection can have on your body. The truth is, if left untreated, infections have the potential to spread to other areas of your body or cause significant problems in the area that it is located. Since bacterial vaginosis is an infection of your vagina, the areas that would be the most greatly affected are your reproductive organs.

If you are of childbearing age and plan on having children one day or more children than what you have now; it is important that you be able to quickly recognize a bacterial vaginosis infection and know how to properly treat it. Keeping your body healthy includes keep it free of infection.

Increases Chance of Contracting Diseases

If having bacterial vaginosis wasn't bad enough, having this infection can also leave you open to contracting other infections and even diseases. While there may be more than what are included in this list, the following diseases and infections are the ones that you are most at risk of catching during a bacterial vaginosis infection:

Pelvic Inflammatory Disease

This is an infection of the uterus and fallopian tubes that, if left untreated, can lead to infertility. If that wasn't enough damage, it could also cause you to have an ectopic pregnancy, if you were to become pregnant while infected. This can be life threatening if your fallopian tube bursts from the growth of the embryo.

Sexually Transmitted Diseases /Infections

Having Bacterial Vaginosis leaves you more susceptible to catching STDs such as chlamydia, gonorrhea, HPV and herpes. Just like pelvic inflammatory disease, leaving these diseases, (specifically chlamydia and gonorrhea), untreated can lead to infertility while HPV can lead to cervical cancer. As for herpes, that is an infection that you may keep with you for the rest of your life as it cannot be easily cured.

HIV

As you probably know, HIV is the virus that causes AIDS. This is the one virus that you absolutely do not want to get because if it transforms into AIDS, there is no cure and it is often fatal. In addition, if a woman has both bacterial vaginosis and AIDS, she is much more likely to pass the virus on to her partner.

Post-Surgery Infection

Any surgery such as a hysterectomy or abortion while you are infected with bacterial vaginosis can lead to additional infection in the site of the surgery. One of the biggest risks of surgery is infection. So if you add in the increased risk of already having an infection that could spread, this could potentially leave you with a more difficult and longer recovery time. In fact, many physicians recommend that before any such surgery, women should be treated for bacterial vaginosis just in case they have it.

In general, if you have an infection somewhere in your body then your overall immunity is lower than normal. This could leave you susceptible to colds and other airborne viruses. If your good bacteria have been overcome by bad bacteria, then it is that much harder for them to fight off the bad bacteria. Infection will also leave your white blood count low, which also leaves your body with a lower defense in case of a virus attack. This will also allow more viruses in and can take you longer to fight them off.

It Can Negatively Affect Your Pregnancy

Being pregnant should be a wonderful time. Many women do their best to stay healthy during their pregnancy so that they can have a healthy delivery. They avoid being around people that are sick and stay away from medications that could be harmful to their unborn baby. Unfortunately, despite their best efforts, they can still end up with a bad case of bacterial vaginosis.

In fact, pregnant women are at an increased risk of catching bacterial vaginosis. When you are pregnant, your body is going through major changes that often spur the onset of bacterial vaginosis such as an increased hormone level, extra discharge that leaves your vaginal area extra moist and even being more prone to catching it from sexual activity.

If you do end up with bacterial vaginosis, it usually doesn't increase your risk of complications during pregnancy but like everything else, it can present some risks such as:

Preterm Delivery

Just having the infection can cause you to give birth to your baby earlier than full time. Pre-term babies often have a low birth weight and lungs that are not fully developed. If this happens, your baby will have to stay hospitalized longer than usual, may have developmental delays or even death.

Late Miscarriage

Many miscarriages occur in the first trimester of pregnancy- often before a woman even realizes she is pregnant. However, if you have bacterial vaginosis, you have a greater chance of miscarrying in the second or third trimester of your pregnancy. If you are nearing the end of your pregnancy, it can also result in giving birth to a stillborn baby.

Ruptured Amniotic Sac

Complications from the infection can cause the amniotic sac to rupture. If this happens, this could result in anything from being put on bed rest, premature delivery miscarriage or stillborn birth.

Chorioamnionitis

This condition is when the membranes surrounding the fetus become inflamed. This can cause your child to be born preterm which means that they baby may not survive. If the baby does survive, it can be left with a condition called cerebral palsy.

Postpartum endometritis

After giving birth, the lining of your uterus can get irritated and even inflamed. This can lead to shedding more of the lining and thus bleeding heavier.

Tubal Factor Infertility

If you are not pregnant yet but are trying to become pregnant, if you have a prolonged bacterial vaginosis infection, you can end up with fallopian tube damage which can make it impossible for an egg to make it to the uterus to be fertilized, thus making you infertile.

In vitro Fertilization

If you are trying to become pregnant through in vitro fertilization, your success rate of becoming pregnant is significantly reduced if you have bacterial vaginosis.

When it comes to your pregnancy, you don't want any more risks or complications than you already have. A healthy pregnancy and resulting baby should always be your focus. Even if you aren't planning to get pregnant, accidents happen, so you really want to make sure that you take all the precautions that you can to keep from developing bacterial vaginosis. This includes making sure you are free of the infection before you get pregnant in the first place.

Limits the Things You Can Do

When you look at all the effects that bacterial vaginosis can have on your body, it should be enough for you to want to get rid of bacterial vaginosis for good. However, bacterial vaginosis's grip on your life goes way beyond the physical effects.

A bacterial vaginosis infection has the great ability of ruining almost everything that you used to enjoy. It may seem a bit dramatic to say this but if you really think about, it affects many activities of your daily life.

Sex

The first and most obvious is sex. Even if you have been married to the same man for years, if you have a bacterial vaginosis infection you will be too embarrassed to have sex. This is for the most part because the fishy smell is overbearing. In fact, the smell only intensifies during sex. This is not only a turn off for the women, but sad to say it can be a real turn off to a man. This is the main reason while women will refrain from sex while infected

Another reason that bacterial vaginosis will keep you from sex is because of the pain that it causes. Upon penetration you can experience a stinging or burning pain so uncomfortable that you may skip sex altogether. As you know, if you are in a long term relationship, skipping sex for a period of time can really put a strain on your relationship. In fact, it can take a lot of the romance and desire right out of your relationship.

Swimming

Whether it is swimming in a swimming pool, the ocean or a lake, having bacterial vaginosis can keep you from doing it. This goes back to the whole embarrassment issue, because of the foul smell. After all, if you are wearing just a swim suit, that doesn't give you too much coverage. The possibility that others will be able to smell it is enough to keep you out of the water.

Another reason is because the excess discharge can make you feel unclean. The thought of discharge making contact with the water (as it inevitably will) is not only unhygienic but also just plain gross. Even your nightly soaking in your bathtub may be out of the question for you.

Going to the Gym

If you have a bacterial vaginosis infection, you probably will have no interest in getting undressed in front of anyone else, even if it is just in the locker room in the gym. You will be worried that a wafting odor may be smelled by others or maybe the infection just keeps you feeling extra sensitive around others.

Furthermore, you might not want to use a piece of exercise equipment that others are waiting to use ,out of fear that you may leave an odor behind and then they will know that it came from you. Another thing to consider is that if you start sweating, your underwear may become even more wet and uncomfortable.

Going Shopping

That's right, even your favorite pastime can be affected by having bacterial vaginosis. When you are not feeling clean in that area, it can make you nervous about leaving a smell or even discharge on clothes that you are trying on. Furthermore, trying on pants can really cause discomfort as you pull them on and off. As a matter of fact, even just walking around the stores can be uncomfortable for you if your pants are too tight, thus causing you to itch or if the moistness of your underwear gets to be too much.

Anything else that you can think of can be affected by bacterial vaginosis. It could be because of the sheer discomfort that the infection causes, or due to the embarrassment that you feel because of it. Bacterial vaginosis can make you feel dirty and even gross. It seems that no matter how often you clean yourself, the odor just comes back and the discharge keeps coming.

You Could be Losing Vitamin B and Folic Acid

If you keep getting bacterial vaginosis then you are probably losing the stored amounts of Vitamin B and folic acid that your body has. Vitamin B is important because it helps to regulate our energy levels. If your level of Vitamin B is low, you will feel tired and weak and will have foggy thinking. In fact, if your levels are too low, you could feel dizzy or too tired to function.

Folic acid on the other hand is important for women of childbearing years to have high levels of. This is the supplement that can help newly forming embryos to develop correctly and also reduces the risk of defects. In fact, most women cannot consume enough of this nutrient through diet alone; so doctors recommend taking a folic acid supplement.

With all this being said, our bodies cannot afford to lose any vitamin B or folic acid. If you feel as though you have a bacterial vaginosis infection, it is wise to start taking vitamin B and folic acid supplements even before you feel that you may be losing these nutrients. (By the way, a good multi-vitamin will provide both these nutrients and it is always a good idea to take them whether you are sick or not).

It's Just a Plain Inconvenience

To top it all off, having a bacterial vaginosis infection is just a pain in the butt (almost literally!). Let's be honest: no one wants to have to deal with an infection. Period! It is not easy to cure it for good. So, you really have to make an effort to change your lifestyle which, no one wants to do.

Also, it makes you change a lot of things you have planned. If you have a date, you may have to delay it a few weeks. If you were supposed to go to the beach with your friends, you may have to delay that for a few weeks. If you have almost anything planned, you will either have to delay it or modify it somehow.

Another annoyingly inconvenient thing about having bacterial vaginosis is that you have to bring extra pairs of underwear with you almost everywhere you go. The discharge can keep you always feeling slimy and unclean so if you don't want to use a panty liner, you will probably feel the need to change into clean underwear every time.

Don't forget about the itching. The itching feeling you get from bacterial vaginosis is not the kind of itch that is relieved once it is scratched. In fact, you can scratch away for 5 minutes and still have the itch afterward. And, the itch is so intense that at times it can be almost impossible to resist scratching. This can lead to yet another source of embarrassment. Imagine if you are sitting at your desk at work when the urge to scratch comes: you start scratching your vaginal area when a co-worker or even your boss walks by and sees you. How about if you are on a date when you start scratching yourself and your date sees you. This is probably one of the most embarrassing things that you could be caught doing in front of someone.

So what do you do? Run to the bathroom every time you have an itch? First of all, you may not make it there in time before you instinctively start scratching but also, what will people think if you are constantly running to the bathroom every few minutes? You won't be able to get all your work done at your job and you most certainly can't have a successful date this way.

This chapter may have been hard to read especially if you have just gotten your first bacterial vaginosis infection and didn't know what to expect. There is no sugar coating this: it is unpleasant and unrelenting. Just when you think it has finally gone away, slowly the symptoms creep back in.

The only way to get rid of it for good is to treat it but that doesn't necessarily mean that you need a doctor. Let's go to the next chapter to find out why.

Chapter 3: Modern Medicine Isn't Always Best

What do you do when you wake up with a fever, cough or any other symptom of being sick? Most likely, you call up your doctor's office and make an appointment to see him or her. Most of the time, we don't even wait to see if the symptoms clear up on their own ,within a few hours, before we rush in to see the doctor.

Modern medicine has come a long way from the medicine men from a few centuries ago; however, doctors aren't miracle workers. Don't get me wrong, if you are truly sick or hurt, your best option is to go straight to your doctor for a diagnosis and treatment if necessary, but as a whole, our society has become entirely too dependent on doctors.

I want to preface this chapter by saying that I in no way am anti-doctor or anti-modern medicine. However, I do believe that sometimes your best treatment is done without your doctor. Let me break this down so that it makes sense:

Why Do You Go To The Doctor?

Really think about this question: why do you go to the doctor? I bet 99% of you will answer "to get better". While this isn't necessarily the wrong answer, it also shouldn't be your first answer. The truth is, in order to stay at your healthiest, you should visit your doctor at the very least on a yearly basis. Prevention is the key to living a healthy and long life. So getting your blood drawn, blood pressure checked and other routine tests is a good thing because it can catch many problems before they even have a chance to materialize.

However, going to the doctor for every sniffle and cough is not necessary. Understanding the human body is a science; a science that is ever changing. At the same time, your doctor is not all knowing. We all would like to believe that if we went to the doctor with an ailment, that our doctor would know what it was immediately and that they would know how to treat it. However, this is not always the case especially when many illnesses have the same symptoms.

Without definitive testing, your doctor's diagnosis is often their best guess based on your symptoms and the likelihood of you being susceptible to a certain disease. Sometimes they are right and can treat you effectively but sometimes they are wrong. Even more importantly, sometimes an illness requires no medical attention at all because it will naturally run its course and be gone. In this case, going to the doctor and taking medicine can only complicate the situation.

Another unfortunate factor is that doctors can occasionally seem quite judgmental. They could jump to conclusions and think that you sleep around because of your bacterial vaginosis condition. They may feel the need to lecture you on safe sex and make you feel embarrassed, especially if you are in a monogamous relationship or are definitely not promiscuous.

Some doctors really don't care whether your symptoms go away or not and so they just prescribe you an antibiotic and send you on your way. If you don't have a life threatening condition, they merely try to make you happy and nothing more. Many even write prescriptions when it isn't necessary, just to appease the patient, which more doctors than you probably think, actually do.

The fact of the matter is that you go to the doctor to find out what is wrong with you and to help you get better because we, as a society, are conditioned into believing that is the way it works. And for the most part, it does. However, a little self-knowledge goes a long way. As long as you know what you are doing, you can skip visiting the doctor and treat bacterial vaginosis on your own - and guess what? You can do a better job at curing it and keeping it from coming back than your doctor could!

The symptoms that you experience from an infection or other illness are not only your body's response to the attack on your body, but also your body's way of letting you know, that something is wrong. If you notice that your vaginal discharge has changed color, consistency or has a foul odor, you should immediately know that something is wrong. The same goes for extreme itching. It is normal to have itchiness sometimes on the outside of your vagina because it could just be contact dermatitis from something you wore or came into contact with. A hive may accompany it and should go away by cleaning the area or using an anti-itch cream. However, if the itching is almost unbearable and is so intense that just your pants rubbing against your vaginal area is uncomfortable, then there is a problem. Finally, if you ever experience vaginal pain during sex or when urinating, this is another indicator from your body that something is wrong.

Your body can present any or even all of these symptoms as a warning that your body is infected with bacterial vaginosis. Now keep in mind that the fact that I am saying that you can handle bacterial vaginosis better than your doctor doesn't mean that you should just sit back and wait for the infection to take its course; it doesn't work that way. Even if the symptoms seem to clear up on their own, you can be assured that bacterial vaginosis is still in your system but just taking a break before showing up again - and, next time, it will be a lot worse.

If you know that you have bacterial vaginosis, then you must take proactive steps to cure it. And, no, this does not mean by taking antibiotics or any other prescribed medication. (This will be discussed in detail in a later chapter.)

Cash Weighs Heavy in Their Diagnosis

It may be hard to believe, but all of the decisions that your doctors make with regard to your health care are not entirely based on your wellbeing. It may seem more than a bit unethical but your treatment options in part are influenced by money. That's right; the money you pay and the money the doctors make all tie in with how much the drug companies make.

Let me explain. First of all, your doctor won't listen to your symptoms over the phone even if it is just a runny nose and a cough. No, they want you to come in instead of saying that you just have a common cold over the phone. One reason for this is because there could be an underlying symptom that you don't recognize which could mean that you have something more advanced than a common cold. This reason is completely understandable.

However, the other big reason is because once you walk through that office door for an appointment, you will be paying a co-pay. Your doctor may even recommend that you return for a follow up appointment in a week or two to make sure that your illness has gone away. Guess what that means? That's right, another co-pay to be paid out of your own pocket and directly into their wallet.

Even more, they will take the office visit as an opportunity to write you out a prescription or two. Like a good patient, you follow your doctor's medical advice and go to the pharmacy to fill your prescription(s). Now the pharmaceutical companies are profiting from your illness, too.

Never thought of it that way? Many people don't. This is because you usually start to feel better after taking the medicine - not because it is curing you, but because the natural course of your cold or other virus has run its natural course. So you go on to believe that you made the right decision to go to the doctor because you needed the medication to get better.

The truth is, many times you don't even need to step into the doctor's office in order to get better. Even more times, you don't even need the medicine that was prescribed to you in order to get better. The medical industry is a business after all, and you should always remember the goal of every business - to make money.

Does Your Doctor Know How to Treat Bacterial Vaginosis?

If you have a vaginal infection, you don't want to go to your general doctor unless they perform pap smears in their office on a regular basis. You are better off going to your gynecologist who is very familiar with the reproductive system and its correlating diseases and infections. After all, if you had a heart condition, would you go to your primary doctor or would you go to a cardiologist who actually specializes in the heart and conditions that affect it?

If you have had bacterial vaginosis before and are sure that is what you have, then you may not even have to go to the doctor to be diagnosed. However, if this is your first bacterial vaginosis infection, it is a good idea to go to your gynecologist to confirm that this is actually what you have. Like I said before, there are so many other vaginal infections that have the same or similar symptoms that it is easy to get it confused. This includes, yeast infections and even some sexually transmitted diseases. If you treat yourself based on your own diagnosis, and are wrong, then the real problem won't be solved.

Many infections and diseases can lead to further complications including the infection spreading and causing even infertility. That's why it is so important to verify that you actually have bacterial vaginosis in the first place and not something else. Your doctor will use a swab or plastic loop to take a sample of the cells from the wall of your vagina and send it to the lab. There the sample will be put under a microscope to see if there are any organisms typical of bacterial vaginosis present. They look specifically for clue cells which are vaginal lining cells that have organisms' specific to bacterial vaginosis.

When the test comes back from the lab, your doctor will call you and let you know whether it is bacterial vaginosis or another type of infection. At this point, your doctor will try to prescribe you an antibiotic. But if it is bacterial vaginosis that you are infected with, an antibiotic will not do you much good. It will only give you some temporary relief, and your doctor knows it.

Now don't get me wrong; your doctor is not going out of his way to hurt you just to make a few extra bucks. In fact, your doctor probably believes that he is helping you by giving you brief relief from your symptoms and even giving you some piece of mind. But he also knows that you will soon be back to see him when the symptoms return. But this doesn't bother him, because he knows this means more money in his pocket. Anyway, by giving you the prescription, you can't come back and say that he did nothing to try to help you. At this point, he will just write you another prescription for a yet another, stronger antibiotic. Of course, you will return to his office once again when your symptoms return, and then it is a never-ending cycle of improper treatment and more money being paid to the doctor and pharmaceutical companies.

Avoid this pointless cycle by passing on the antibiotic. If you feel weird telling your doctor that you don't want an antibiotic or if you are a little leery that you cannot heal this infection on your own, then take the prescription but don't fill it. Having it as a backup may give you some piece of mind but remember it will do you no good in the long run.

Our next chapter will tell you exactly why you should refuse an antibiotic to treat your bacterial vaginosis infection and how it can really do you more harm than good.

Chapter 4: Getting Rid of It Without Antibiotics

Science has come a long way. In this day and age, we have a cure for a larger number of infections and diseases - far more than we had a century ago, or even a decade ago for that matter. If you stop to think about it, modern medicine is pretty amazing. How do they come up with the right cure to the right disease?

For the most part, it is all about trial and error. They try out different compounds until one seems to be effective for a certain disease. However, everyone's body reacts differently to each and every medicine. After all, medicine isn't made to treat you and your body specifically; it is a one size fits all kind of deal. Therefore, the medicine that should get rid of your infection may leave you with a host of other problems. Another thing to consider is that many medicines are still fairly new. So, all the side effects that could be caused by them years down the road are still not even known yet.

Nonetheless, antibiotics are still prescribed over and over again. Antibiotics are typically effective in about 90% of cases where they are correctly prescribed for bacterial vaginosis. However, out of this 90%, 25% of women will end up battling bacterial vaginosis again, in less than just four weeks. So why do doctors keep prescribing antibiotics if they aren't a real cure and why should you avoid them? Hopefully, I can explain this to you in this chapter.

Typical Prescriptions Given to Treat Bacterial Vaginosis

If you go to the doctor with symptoms of bacterial vaginosis, your doctor will typically prescribe you an antibiotic whether it is proven that you have the infection or not. The doctor may not even acknowledge whether you have bacterial vaginosis or not, because he may be unsure himself, but he may still prescribe an antibiotic "just in case". So you can be prepared with some knowledge. These are the antibiotics most usually prescribed to treat bacterial vaginosis:

Metronidazole

This medication is typically taken orally two times a day for seven days, although it is sometimes prescribed to be taken only once instead, for the seven days. If directed to take this pill just once, bacterial vaginosis is much more likely to return. It is also sometimes prescribed in gel form to be applied one time a day, for five days. Don't be confused by the gel form - it is still a prescription.

Clindamycin

This is a stronger antibiotic which is usually prescribed when metronidazole doesn't clear up the infection or if the bacterial vaginosis comes back again (which it will). It can either be dispensed as a vaginal cream to be applied one time a day for a week or in pill form though this isn't as common anymore because it presents a big risk of developing *pseudomembranous colitis* among other things.

Tinidazole

Similar to clindamycin, tinidazole is typically prescribed if metronidazole doesn't work or if bacterial vaginosis resurfaces. This antibiotic is taken as a single dose in a pill form. However, you cannot consume any alcohol while on this antibiotic.

Antibiotics Can Do More Harm Than Good

Antibiotics are a great medical invention. There are some infections that cannot be cured without their help. A great example of Strep Throat comes to mind. Without treating this infection, the bacteria will spread and your heart will be affected. Though your symptoms might clear up for a few days or even weeks, you can't be fooled into thinking that it is gone away on its own. The infection is actually just lying dormant. When the symptoms re-appear, they will typically be much worse than the first time and can start to do some real damage. Penicillin has been proven to get rid of this infection for good, at least until you are re-exposed to strep throat again.

In that case, antibiotics will usually do more good than harm (although there are always exceptions to the rule). This is because if properly diagnosed through a positive strep test, the need of an antibiotic is absolute. Without it, your body will go through a lot of pain and even damage. So even if you do experience typical side effects of antibiotics, the good outweighs the bad.

However, there are many cases where antibiotics do more harm than good. The first reason is that antibiotics are over prescribed. We all have learned by exposure that your doctor knows what is best for you and that there is no reason to question your doctor. In reality, you should always question your doctor. This is not to say that your doctor is out to get you or to hurt you, but rather, that there are a few reasons why a doctor will prescribe an antibiotic, even though it isn't necessary:

To make the patient happy

The number one reason that a doctor will prescribe an antibiotic even though it is not medically necessary is to appease the patient. For the most part, a patient comes in to see the doctor because they are sick or think they may have an infection. They expect to be given a prescription to treat the problem. If a doctor says that that there is nothing that they can give them to clear it up or that it will clear up on its own, some patients get upset.

They either think that an antibiotic will help clear it up quicker or worry that they will only get worse and then have to return to the doctor. Many like to have the prescription "just in case" the infection or illness doesn't go away. The doctor basically just wants to shut the patient up or doesn't want them to complain; so they prescribe them an antibiotic even if they know the patient doesn't need it.

To make the drug companies happy

It's a sad fact but the drug companies have a lot more say when it comes to your treatment than you think. Drug company reps visit doctors at their office on a regular basis to promote their brand of drugs. They also push doctors to write prescriptions for these drugs over others.

Many doctors listen to these reps because they get many free samples, free tickets and even free meals. So doctors will write out prescriptions in exchange for what the drug reps are offering them in exchange. Because of this, they usually have no qualms about prescribing an antibiotic that isn't necessary for your condition.

To make himself happy

Some doctors will write you a prescription for an antibiotic even though you don't need it just for their own sake. Perhaps they believe they have an ethical obligation to offer some sort of treatment, no matter what you're suffering from. Others worry, that if your condition changes and they never prescribed you anything, they could face a medical malpractice suit. Others write the prescription for you to have "just in case".

No matter the reason, doctors are doing you a disservice by writing you a prescription for an antibiotic that they know you do not need.

We Are Building a Resistance Against Antibiotics

Even if you are prescribed an appropriate antibiotic to treat an infection, antibiotics are not always effective. Although one reason could be that everyone's body responds to each drug differently, there is a bigger reason: people do not follow the directions. Take this as an example: you are given an antibiotic to treat strep throat with the prescribed dose as 4 pills per day for 10 days. You take the antibiotic exactly as prescribed for the first 3 days. By the fourth day, you feel a lot better and miss a couple of doses. By day 7 you feel 100% better so you stop taking the antibiotic because you feel that you are healed.

This is a big no-no. Even though your symptoms are gone, it doesn't mean that the infection is entirely gone from your body. This can lead to two things: one, the infection will return shortly thereafter; and two, you are building a resistance against the antibiotic. Either scenario will open your body up to more infection. If the strep throat comes back a couple weeks later, it may be even worse than the first time. If you start to build a resistance towards the antibiotic, it will either not be as effective in your treatment or won't be effective at all.

For some reason, people tend to view antibiotics much differently than other prescribed medication such as pain killers. You probably realize that if you use a pain killer too often or differently as directed, then you can build a resistance to it. You will either need a higher dose or a different drug all together to alleviate your pain. I'm sure you are careful to take these types of prescriptions as closely as prescribed as possible.

However, when it comes to antibiotics, people seem to have no problem shortening their treatment on their own and even self-diagnosing. The truth is that antibiotics should be treated as seriously as other prescriptions. If you were able to take antibiotics at your own leisure, then they wouldn't need a prescription - they would be available over the counter.

Antibiotics are Being Overused

Every time I over hear someone talking to another person about how they don't feel well or that they have a cold and the other person responds "maybe you should go to the doctor and get an antibiotic, just in case" it makes me cringe. The number one reason that antibiotics are becoming more and more ineffective is because Americans, as a whole, are overusing them.

Your next question may be "but if you have an infection and are using an antibiotic to clear it up, how is it overuse if it is needed?" Well, first of all, as discussed earlier, people are using antibiotics for reasons other than that it is necessary. You need to understand that antibiotics were created in order to combat certain types of bacterial infections. What this means is that an antibiotic will do absolutely nothing to fight off a virus. Many of the illnesses we get, such as a common cold and even those 24 hour bugs, are caused by viruses. These types of illnesses just have to run their course naturally and cannot be assisted by an antibiotic.

Furthermore, just because you have a bacterial infection doesn't mean that you need an antibiotic to fight it off; such is the case of bacterial vaginosis. Now, this doesn't mean it will naturally run its course and be out of your system either. This just means that you can get rid of the bacterial infection by using other, natural methods that won't harm you in the process, unlike antibiotics.

This gross overuse and misuse of antibiotics is resulting in the creation of more and more "superbugs". These infections are drug resistant and are very hard to get rid of. The condition is so serious that schools have in recent years been shut down and kids have been quarantined when one student is found to have it. One particular strand called MRSA is just one example.

At the rate we are going with antibiotic use, we are going to run into a point when a common illness is going to be entirely resistant to drugs and we are going to enter a plague-like era. These infections are mutating because they have become resistant to the antibiotics used to treat them. Had the antibiotics been used properly in the first place, we would not have this problem and these infections would remain treatable.

They Cause Their Own Side Effects

If an antibiotic is necessary to treat your ailment, its use, will still leave behind some pretty awful side effects. In the case of bacterial vaginosis, using antibiotics can cause a whole slew of new side effects. Sometimes the side effects aren't as bad as the symptoms from the infection, but sometimes they are worse.

By far, the worst side effect of antibiotics is that your immune system will be compromised. While the antibiotic is attacking the bad bacteria, it inadvertently attacks your good bacteria, as well. This means that you end up depleting a great deal of the good bacteria that your body uses to fight off the bad. You will then be more susceptible to other infections and illnesses. Just when you fight off one infection, another one could follow a week later. Of course, the new infection could just be a reoccurrence of the one you thought you had just fought off.

As a matter of fact, this is often the case with bacterial vaginosis. Since it is a chronic condition, you cannot simply take an antibiotic and think that you have been cured. This infection will almost always come back. Think of it this way: antibiotics work by killing bad bacteria while also killing good bacteria, leaving your good bacteria levels low. Now, since bacterial vaginosis is caused when the bad bacteria outnumber the good bacteria in your vagina, doesn't it make sense that if you don't have the normal amount of good bacteria left in your vagina that the bad bacteria can easily overtake them again? The answer is yes, and you are left with yet another bout of bacterial vaginosis.

Two other infections that are a common result of treating your bacterial vaginosis are urinary tract infections and yeast infections. And since they have very similar symptoms as bacterial vaginosis; it will be like it never went away.

If you absolutely must take an antibiotic, you should always also take probiotics. A probiotic is a supplement in pill form that is jam packed with healthy bacteria. In fact, one pill can pack thousands of bacteria. It sounds like a gross concept, willingly letting in thousands upon thousands of bacteria a day. But these are the bacteria that will fight off the bad. In essence, taking probiotics, while on a regime of antibiotics, is like immediately replacing the good bacteria that are being killed by the antibiotic. This will keep your immune system up and help keep you from becoming infected with secondary infections.

Another side effect of taking antibiotics, and also a warning that your good bacteria level is low, is bad breath. This is caused by the healthy bacteria in our intestinal tract being depleted. These bacteria help digest our food so if there aren't enough, it can leave our food only partially digested which means that anything that isn't digested will decay. The foul odor that it produces comes up and out of our mouth.

Other Factors to Consider

Even if you are taking an antibiotic exactly as it was prescribed, it still can be ineffective. There are certain medications such as prescription birth control that when used in conjunction with the antibiotics, can lower its effectiveness. When two conflicting drugs are in your system, the stronger one will win out, rendering the other ineffective. However, it can also lower the effectiveness of both drugs.

Taking antibiotics can cause some real issues with your digestive system. They can do anything from giving you a bad case of diarrhea to making you extremely constipated. They can also make you sick in your stomach and unable to keep your food down. This is due to the fact that they mess with the natural intestinal flora that we all have. These are the bacteria that help keep our digestive system running as it should.

In the end, if you chose to treat your bacterial vaginosis with antibiotics, you may end up with some temporary relief, but it is never a "cure". This is not just my assertion, but rather scientifically proven (remember it is "osis", i.e. chronic) that bacterial vaginosis is a condition that will keep coming back.

The only way to clear it up for good is by making the proper changes that will make your body less susceptible to it. Sorry, but taking antibiotics, is just not part of the changes you need to make.

The changes that you should be making to your body will help you to balance out the bacteria in your vagina and the rest of your body so that your body can naturally heal from bacterial vaginosis.

Let's go to our next and final chapter to find out exactly how to get rid of bacterial vaginosis for good.

Chapter 5: Keeping It Away For Good

So here you are; you know for sure that you have bacterial vaginosis and now you also know that antibiotics won't cure you. At this point, you may be wondering if this is a sham or maybe even that this is just some naturalist's earth-loving agenda. Let me assure you that it is neither.

I understand the frustration, discomfort and embarrassment that bacterial vaginosis puts you through. I also know that the temporary relief that antibiotics can provide just isn't enough. But do you want to know what the best thing I know is? Simply put, it is how to cure it for good without getting into the never ending cycle of doctors and antibiotics.

The Best Cure is Natural: The beatBV^{tm} Cure

When you hear about a cure that is both natural and herbal, you are probably pretty skeptical. Again, this is a product of our societal conditioning that science has the best medicine to cure us. Remember, a few centuries back we didn't have what we have now, including antibiotics. How do you think infection was cured back then? Sure there were diseases that you would die from back then that we now have the cure for; but not every infection and disease is fatal. More importantly, not everything must be cured with an antibiotic or other modern medicine.

Don't worry; I'm not going to tell you to go to an herb store or collect some hard to find plants to use. Instead, I'm going to be focusing on items that you do not need a prescription for along with vitamins and supplements. All you need to do is walk into a multi-purpose store to find these items.

Hydrogen Peroxide

If you want to get rid of the worst bacterial vaginosis symptoms - the itching, discharge and foul smell - you can do so in just a few minutes. All you need is hydrogen peroxide and distilled water to give yourself some immediate discomfort. Yes, it is that simple!

Mix ¼ of a cup of **3% hydrogen peroxide** with ¼ of a cup of distilled water. It is important that you choose **only 3% hydrogen peroxide** because any stronger will be too much for the sensitive skin of your vagina. Likewise, choose distilled water to ensure that you are using pure water without any added chemicals, unlike tap water that contains more than just water.

Use a douche, or any other sanitized container that will work. Insert the mixture into your vagina while lying on your back with your knees up, so it doesn't immediately leak back out. If you notice any white foaming, that means that the hydrogen peroxide is fighting the bad bacteria. Unlike antibiotics, the good bacteria will not be killed, meaning your immune system won't be compromised as a result of this treatment.

After about 5 minutes, get up and rinse out your vagina with just distilled water, nothing else. Then, prepare another mixture of hydrogen peroxide and distilled water and repeat the process. You should immediately feel relief from the itching along with a dryer, cleaner feeling. This will also eliminate the strong fishy odor. Make sure you use this mixture two times a day for a minimum of three days straights. If you notice that the symptoms are still showing up then use for another two days to finish it off.

Lactobacillus Acidophilus

Although the hydrogen peroxide and distilled water mixture is a great way to kill the bad bacteria in your vagina and get relief from the symptoms, it is not enough to keep bacterial vaginosis away for good. In order to keep it from coming back, you have to keep your good bacteria levels high. This good bacterium is called lactobacillus acidophilus.

You can think of good bacteria as soldiers. They are there to protect your body from intruders. If you do not have enough soldiers when the enemy attacks, they will be outnumbered and overcome. In order to make sure that your soldiers can fight off an attack, you need to add more to the army. It makes sense, right?

It used to be common for women suffering with an infection to spoon yogurt into their vagina. Okay, maybe common isn't the right word since you probably have never heard of anyone doing that. Anyway, they would do this because yogurt is known to be packed with good bacteria. By inserting it into your vagina, you were absorbing these good bacteria immediately. However, since it is a rather messy and seemingly unsanitary method, the better option is to take a lactobacillus acidophilus supplement.

It is a pill that you simply swallow with a little bit of water and you are done. When the pills hit your gastrointestinal system, the lactobacillus acidophilus will be absorbed and will boost your amount of good bacteria in your intestinal tract and vagina. If you would rather get the lactobacillus acidophilus straight to the source, there are probiotic inserts that you put directly into our vagina.

Another good thing about lactobacillus acidophilus is that it produces its own natural form of hydrogen peroxide which we already know helps curb your symptoms. These tablets should be applied directly after you have finished your hydrogen peroxide and distilled water cleansing routine.

Folic Acid

Another supplement that will help you to prevent yourself from getting bacterial vaginosis is folic acid. Although you can get this vitamin through some of the foods you eat, it is typically not enough. Therefore, you should take a supplement in pill form. If you would like to increase your intake through foods as well, the following contain high levels of folic acid:

Oranges

Grape fruit

Sprouts

Nuts

Seeds

Beans

Peas

Whole wheat bread

Dark, leafy green vegetables

If you are eating some of the above foods every day along with taking a daily multi-vitamin, you should be getting a great deal of folic acid into your daily diet. However, if you feel as though you won't eat these foods often enough, then you may want to look into a *folic acid supplement*. You might even want to look into using prenatal vitamins because they have very high levels of folic acid - much more than regular multivitamins. Plus, you would still get the benefit of all the other vitamins that you should be taking on a daily basis.

Change Your Diet

It was discussed earlier how toxins in our food can negatively impact your immune system and your susceptibility to infections and illness. Therefore, if you change your diet to eliminate most of these toxins you can subsequently lower your risk of infection and illness.

What we eat and drink is directly correlated to just about everything that has to do with our bodies. Besides improving our overall health and boosting our immune system, a healthy diet can also do everything from increasing our energy levels to clear blemishes. It only makes sense that something that is so vital to us staying alive would have such an impact on every other aspect of our lives, too.

Water

You cannot survive long without drinking water. In fact, just a few hours without water will negatively impact your body. Water helps nutrients to reach every cell of your body. It is necessary for digestion, circulation and to keep your excretory system functioning. In addition, it helps to regulate your body temperature so that it doesn't get too high.

The fact is that many of us are not drinking enough water on a daily basis. Even if you drink some when you get thirsty, it is not enough. Here's why: by the time you are thirsty, you are already dehydrated. Therefore, if you make sure that you are drinking enough water through the day, you will not feel thirsty. Feeling thirsty is your body's first warning to you that you are dehydrated but you can avoid this by staying properly hydrated.

The rule of thumb is that you need *8 glasses of water a day in order to stay properly hydrated.* However, depending on your size you may need more than 64 ounces a day. Try drinking an 8 ounce glass every 2 hours that you are awake and you should be able to meet your 8 glasses a day goal. Keep in mind that if you are exercising or doing any other strenuous activity, you will need to drink even more water in order to stay hydrated. Remember, when you sweat, you are losing water so you must replace it.

If you find it difficult to get in 8 glasses of water a day, sit back and think about what else you are drinking during the day. Drinking coffee, soda and juice won't leave you much room for water. Try to limit your coffee to one cup in the morning and eliminate soda and sweetened juices entirely. Not only do they have you consuming hundreds of extra calories a day but they are also pretty much void of any nutritional content. Instead of filling up on drinks that will not benefit you any, stick to water instead.

Food

Food is a major problem in America these days. All you have to do is look at statistics that show that *1/3 of people in this country (that's 1 out of every 3 people!) are overweight* in order to see that there is a problem. We didn't see this problem 50 years ago. In fact, we didn't have such a massive problem 20 years ago. We can blame this fairly new epidemic on food. Manufacturers are trying to make food appeal even more to people, especially children, by filling it with extra fatty ingredients. They hope that if they make these foods irresistible, that consumers will buy more and more. They have no regard to the health of those eating their product; they only care about making more money.

They add artificial preservatives into products to make them more shelf stable so that they won't go bad before they can be sold (and thus lose money). These artificial preservatives are not healthy for us to consume. They are even adding hormones and other additives to live stock whose meat and milk is then sold to us to consume. This is a fairly new thing made common just about the same time that the obesity rate in kids skyrocketed. Is there a connection between the two? You decide for yourself.

The obesity problem is not just making people fat; it is also increasing health risks such as heart attacks, stroke and other conditions that can be fatal. If the toxins in food have this kind of effect on your body, don't you think it could be infecting our healthy bacteria and thus leaving us more susceptible to infections and diseases including bacterial vaginosis.

Start choosing simpler foods. Generally speaking, *the fewer ingredients a food has, the better it is for you.* Complex carbs and fiber- filled food are not only healthy but also filling. Stop choosing convenience foods and anything labelled "extra" or "loaded". This doesn't mean you have to start counting calories but at least start looking at the nutrition labels on the back of the package to see what exactly you are consuming.

Don't Forget to Get Enough Sleep

Many people really underestimate the importance of sleep. Sleeping is like recharging a battery; without it, you will just fizzle out. Some people get into the habit of sleeping for only 4 or 5 hours a night and believe that they are getting enough sleep because they can function the next day. Others are so busy that they hate "wasting time" on sleep, following the saying "I can sleep when I am dead".

Well the truth of the matter is, no matter how you feel the next day; you should be getting *a minimum of 7 hours of sleep per night. The average amount of sleep that adults need is 8 hours but some people only need 7 while some need 9.* Studies have shown that people that get less sleep than 7-9 hours have a bigger chance of becoming overweight and of having a lower immune system.

Therefore, if you are getting enough sleep on a regular basis, your immune system will get a boost and your chances of catching an illness or infection will be lowered. If you keep getting bacterial vaginosis, take a look at your sleeping habits and make an adjustment.

Try to Relax a Little

People these days seem to always be on the go. They rush to get to work on time, rush home to take care of their home and their families. Between work, school and other activities, you can find yourself burning the candle at both ends. Rest assured that this is not healthy.

Being on the go like this or constantly having a never ending to do list, will keep your stress at an unhealthy level. Stop over committing yourself and take a moment to breathe. Nothing is as important as your health, and if you are too stressed, your health will suffer. If you are constantly stressed out, frazzled or worried about something, your immune system will be lowered; thus leaving you more susceptible to becoming sick. This of course, as you guessed it, includes getting bacterial vaginosis.

If you can't keep your stress level down, no matter what else you are doing, you will eventually get sick. So try to prioritize all the tasks in your life and tackle them one by one. If something doesn't get done - just relax. Spend your time enjoying life instead of worrying about it.

Extra Tips to Avoid Bacterial Vaginosis

In addition to all the information that has already been given, there are a few more things that you can do to protect yourself from getting bacterial vaginosis. They may seem minor but they actually can play a big role in your developing a vaginal infection.

Don't use colored toilet paper

Sure pink toilet paper is pretty but it serves no other special purpose besides looking fancy. The chemicals used to turn the toilet paper pink come into direct contact with your vagina and can irritate you.

Wipe from front to back

I know this may be taking it back to potty training days but remember to always wipe from the front of your vagina, back to your rectum. There are bacteria living in and around your rectum that if presented to your vagina can bring on a serious infection.

Keep your vagina dry

If you go swimming, change out of your wet clothes immediately. Sitting with wet underwear or bathing suit bottoms will only breed bacteria in your vagina leaving you open to infection.

Keep your vagina clean

Simply put, always wear a fresh pair of underwear. Not only should you change into a clean pair every morning, but if you soil them with vaginal discharge, blood or even urine (no matter if it is just a drop), change into a fresh pair immediately.

Don't wear tight underwear or pants

Tight clothing in your vaginal area not only can incite moisture but also keeps your vagina from breathing. Unbleached cotton underwear is best because it allows air to circulate.

Use unscented detergent to clean your underwear

Wash your underwear as naturally as possible. Any perfumes or scented chemicals will just irritate your vagina.

In Conclusion

I know it is hard to believe that an infection like bacterial vaginosis can be treated in ways that seems so simple and easy, and without the help of a doctor or antibiotics. This method of eradicating bacterial vaginosis from your life can not only provide great relief and essentially boost your overall health, but is also basically risk free. You won't lose anything by trying it - and it cannot leave you in worse condition then when you started.

If you are sure that you have bacterial vaginosis, than I urge you to try this method of healing before seeking a prescription from your doctor. If you follow these instructions and you find no relief of the symptoms or see that the infection is still around, then go to the doctor. However, if this is the case, it is a safe bet that it was not bacterial vaginosis but another infection or disease instead.

All that is left for you to do is put this plan into action and start living a life without the discomfort or embarrassment of bacterial vaginosis!

Exclusive Bonus Download: Gluten Free Living Secrets

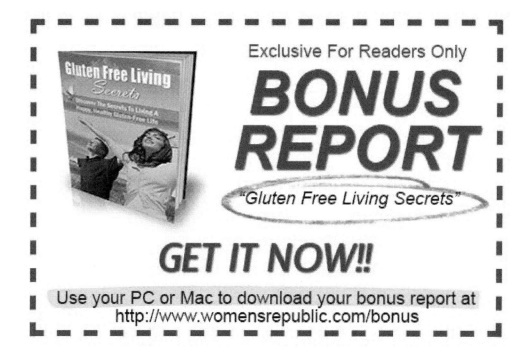

Download your bonus, please visit the download link above from your PC or MAC. To open PDF files, visit http://get.adobe.com/reader/ to download the reader if it's not already installed on your PC or Mac. To open ZIP files, you may need to download WinZip from http://www.winzip.com. This download is for PC or Mac ONLY and might not be downloadable to kindle.

Are you sick and tired of trying every weight loss program out there and failing to see results? Or are you frustrated with not feeling as energetic as you used to despite what you eat? Perhaps you always seem to have a bit of a "dodgy stomach" and indigestion seems to be a regular part of your life?

There's nothing worse than sitting down to a nice big plate of pasta and enjoying your meal only to be met with a growling stomach and the inevitable rush to the toilet.

It's that bloated feeling you get after eating a piece of bread that just "doesn't seem right" . Almost as if you've eaten something poisonous.

Gluten Free Living Secrets is a complete resource that will tell you everything you need to know about the dangers of eating gluten and how to go about transitioning yourself and your family to a life free of this dangerous substance.

Here's just a taste of what you will discover inside Gluten Free Living Secrets:

- What foods you should focus on when first switching to a gluten-free diet

- The 9 grains that are safe and gluten-free

- The truth about whether you can eat pasta on a gluten-free diet

- What you should know to determine if you have Celiac Disease

- and that's not all...

- Why you may want to consider eliminating gluten from your child's diet

- The top 10 reasons to go gluten-free

- How to transform your pantry to be gluten-free

- A list of essential gluten-free shopping tips

- How to keep your kids happy around their gluten-eating friends

- Tips on staying gluten-free when eating out

Gluten Free Living Secrets comes in a digital PDF format that is easy to read either on your computer or on your eBook reader.

Visit the URL above to download this guide and start improving your overall health NOW

One Last Thing...

When you turn the page, Kindle will give you the opportunity to rate the book and share your thoughts on Facebook and Twitter. If you believe the book is worth sharing, would you take a few seconds to let your friends know about it? If it turns out to make a difference in their overall health, they'll be forever grateful to you. As I will.

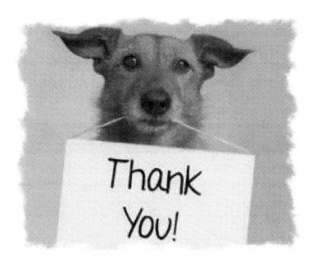

******

Books by This Author:

Permanently Beat Bacterial Vaginosis

Permanently Beat Yeast Infection & Candida

Permanently Beat Urinary Tract Infections

Permanently Beat Hypothyroidism Naturally

Permanently Beat PCOS

The Permanently Beat PCOS Diet & Exercise Shortcuts

The Permanently Beat Hypothyroidism Diet & Exercise Shortcuts

About the Author

Caroline D. Greene is a mother of 2 wonderful girls and a wife to a supportive husband. She has dedicated the past seven years to researching the various women's health topics that are not being openly discussed and providing help and support to the women dealing with these issues in their daily life.

Caroline D. Greene

Published by Women's Republic

Atlanta, Georgia USA

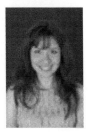

32989310R00024

Printed in Great Britain
by Amazon